FIVE
FUNDAMENTAL
FORCES

D1602259

FIVE FUNDAMENTAL FORCES

Poems

Pattie Palmer-Baker

Pattie Palmer-Baker

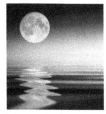

MoonPath Press

Poetry
ISBN 978-1-936657-78-0

Cover art: *Five Fundamental Forces*, collage on paste paper, by Pattie Palmer-Baker

Author photo: Robert R. Sanders (RobertSandersCreative.com)

Book design by Tonya Namura, using Minion Pro.

MoonPath Press, an imprint of Concrete Wolf Poetry Series, is dedicated to publishing the finest poets living in the U.S. Pacific Northwest.

MoonPath Press
PO Box 445
Tillamook, OR 97141

MoonPathPress@gmail.com

http://MoonPathPress.com

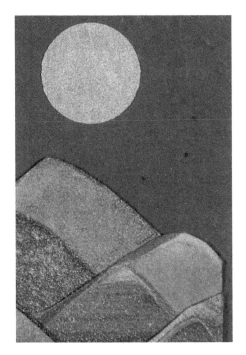

for Kate MacMillan, my beloved sister

Loving anybody and being loved by anybody
is a tremendous danger, a tremendous responsibility.
—James Baldwin

Contents

FIVE
FUNDAMENTAL
FORCES

I. APPLE

A Is for Apple

The one Eve eats,
although God warns her

DO NOT PARTAKE.

The snake all silver sinew and darting gold tongue
says, *yeah, but look how round red shiny and satiny,*
although I am only guessing,
fingerless and toothless as I am.
His lipless mouth curves into a Satan smile.

That first white bite spurts honeyed juice.
In a voice sticky with the apple's syrupy fluid
she says to Adam, *try this.* He salivates
as his hand rounds the forbidden orb.

God roars.
For the first time
thunder and lightning
shatters the azure sky.

The silken tiger bares his eyeteeth
at the rabbit who white-streaks
into trembling shrubs,
at the deer who velvet-leaps
the hedge now sprouting thorns,
at Adam and Eve who stumble-run
into the darkening cooling
forest where they tumble to the ground
no longer pillowed with waiting ferns.

Eve clutches Adam's body
for warmth for comfort.
Love is born.

Abel is killed.

Sixty-Five Million Shades In-Between

white—
piled clouds
frosted maple leaves
yellow-drained winter sunlight
a dying mother's hair white-
whorled on her neck
the eye
of a sixty-five million carat diamond
where the mother curls
around the salt-sculpted father.

black—
sightless sky
rain-slicked slate
coal glittering on buckled rock walls
a black hole sucking in
mother
father
diamonds
white
brown
red
yellow
and sixty-five million shades in-between
even the color of death
cannot escape.

Not Enough Love

My father, one of the first to land
in massacre-ravaged Manilla,
World War II.
His heart roughed up.
By the broken buildings
slumped on their sides leaking
black oil, black smoke, black blood.
By streets choked
insensible with bodies sprawled
on their backs, their stomachs, their sides.
By arms ripped off,
arms that once held
a sister, a husband, a wife, a brother, a baby, a …
By legs cocked
at severe angles, legs that once ran
to catch the bus or walked
to a job hated but with legs that thrummed
with secret gladness for a life
that could stretch 600,000 hours long—
cut short, everything cut short.
Even the dawn of the day.

What else is there to write
about except my mother?
Her sorrow-rinsed gray eyes.
Her smile trembling at her mouth's corner.
How love could not save,
could not patch up,
could not renovate,
my father's heart.

Glitter Love

My momma says, *look at that sunflower!* Taller than me, yellow with a pebbly middle, brown like my daddy's coffee. I reach up to touch the little lumps. Not like rocks. Soft like my white smooth-bumped bedspread. I look down. Much better, the broken glass next to my feet. Every color I love. Red, blue, green, yellow and even diamond-like. The sun explodes the color in each jagged piece. I love anything that glitters.

Morning after morning, my father slips into a plate of glittery glass. His eyes gleam the color of an early morning sky, his crooked smile glints as he tosses out words funny and smart and shiny. My sunflower momma leans on the hard edges. So slim, she sometimes slides in with him. I can't see her, but I know she's in there because yellow-gold flares.

Once at Venice Beach my dad lifted me onto his shoulders and swam us to where the waves lifted and dropped us until I forgot the unmoving land-locked world. The water glimmered navy blue, the foam white-sparkled. That night in bed my body rose and fell on remembered swells of love shimmering.

But. Years later. I can't touch his too soft skin, his too tender heart, his bones too sad. The glass is too resistant. But not diamond hard. Fissures sprout. The glass splinters. My mother squints away the cracks. My eyes, my sister's eyes slide off the crazed surface. No one hears the shatter nor the swallows of brown-gold washing down all those white pills shining in the motel's thick black air. He is dead.

My mother's sunflower petals brush the grieving floor. She is not dead. Her stem straightens. Slowly. Her petals once barely warmed by my father's low level shine reach toward the sky. The sun kisses each one. Now she loves my sister. Now she loves me. Now she feeds her yellow glow to our starving skin.

Ode to Breakfast

Oatmeal mounded with brown sugar, cream skimmed from the bottled milk swirling rivers around a square of centered butter. Eggs fried in bacon grease with yolks softly firm. Scrambled eggs creamy, fluffy. Toast butter-slathered, cinnamon and sugar-dusted. I walk to school. Alone. But with one of those breakfasts settling contentedly within me.

On the weekends, my favorite, crisp deeply buttered, whole wheat toast waits for me in the O'Keefe and Merritt warming drawer. Never soggy, never burned, crisper by the hour until almost friable, crunchy all the way through bites and chews. My mother's loving pale small slightly work-roughened hands, (the last two fingers of her left hand bent and crooked after a truck crashed into the side of her Model A rolling over her hand gripping the top of the car window) situate the toasted bread in the welcoming drawer while I sleep late. Crackly bacon too and that deeply brown toast just for me, well, no, enough for my sister

(who reminds me we did have a third sister
[older]
she tossed me aside when she was nine,
I was five and one half
no longer fun
the good girl
she hated.

I don't know if she ate the toast or bacon or anything
or if she even came out of her bedroom,
she has ghosted my memory).

I do know I cannot find any toast that loved my mouth
the way that toast did.

Devil Doll

While my sister and I roll down
the forever front lawn,
in our bedroom, Crazy Doll murders
our pretty dolls, maims the pretend babies,
bites holes in our biggest teddy bear.
We find her under the bed,
her tufted head turned away,
blue eyes glassed-over.
No use talking to her,
our sentences rock and buckle.
Time to toss her into the closet asylum.

A few weeks later her sobs,
I've changed,
I will never again,
uncurl our rolled-up hearts.
We open the black-filled closet.
Our forgiving hands free her.
Once again, we believe her.
Once again, we forgive her.
Once again Crazy Doll cracks.
Dead dolls litter the floor,
injured ones writhe when we daub
iodine on their open wounds.
Across my lap Crazy Doll spread-eagles.
The closet for the insane
does not a sane doll make,
I say to my little sister,
who rounds her China-blue eyes,
leans close and whispers,
She is a devil-doll.

In the pantry under us,
heavy footfalls break the air.
A cupboard whines open,
the cork squeaks out of a bottle.
Through clenched teeth my sister
squeezes the question,
Is Daddy drinking again?
For a second, I forget how to breathe.
Crazy Doll squirms in my lap,
begs for another chance.
I shake her until her body whiplashes.
No … more … chances!
Off with your head!

Yes, yes, my sister breathes.

Unwhite

My best friend Carmen and I are ten. We walk hand in hand to the public pool even though it's over a mile away in traffic-glutted L.A. These are different times. Guns do not point everywhere shooting anyone, and innocent buildings do not suddenly blow up. Smog usually saturates the atmosphere, but today blue-green and gold stain the air. This is before boys, before questions like *should we diet to get rid of the bit of fat rolling around our waistline, is allowing their tongues to touch ours a mortal sin, should we wear eyeliner inside the eyelid, how oh how do we get boys to want us?* But now we are only ten. The pool awaits us where aquamarine satin will engulf our bodies. We will glide dive dunk splash, we will float, we will skim the surface, and our skin will soften with gladness. Carmen who makes me laugh, who understands me, who loves me, will be my friend forever, and we will never stop trekking to the pool. We will erupt with joy the moment the not too hot not to cold just right water caresses our preadolescent glossy, supple bodies. As time goes on, together we will navigate boys, sex, love, happily ever after. But no, we won't. I turn twelve. I am enrolled in a prestigious private girl's school. Carmen is not. My parents say I can no longer be her friend, Carmen's coffee mocha skin is too brown. The girls attending this painted white school building are milky-white, none are even tan.

Without a Life Vest

My mother makes Christmas pies.
I eat leftover dough baked
with cinnamon sugar butter,
taste my mother's palm prints.

I hold the ribbon
while she ties bows on Christmas presents.
Even though he never says it,
your dad loves you, she says.
Without moving her lips.

At summer's first touch,
I beg for bare feet to race
through sprinklers arcing rainbows.
I shuck shoes on the way
to the beach house. Three weeks—
my mother sweeps sand out the door
reads novels, smokes cigarettes.
I wade in the lacy bones of spent waves,
collect unbroken scallop seashells,
wait for my father's weekend visits.

Sunday morning, he swings
me onto his shoulders, strides
into the heaving ocean.
I stretch my eyes open wide
as we climb water mountains,
plunge down the trenches.
Over and over.

I turn eleven.
He loosens my grip finger by finger,
without a life vest I fall.
I cannot stop falling. He doesn't see.

He looks at my mother
through a bottle of Jim Beam,
smiles a gold watered-down smile.
She fixes her eyes on his drinking mouth,
sometimes spies me from the corner
of her eyes bleeding tears.

The Hand-Off

The speedometer trembles at one-twenty
but the Cadillac runs smooth, silent
as my father steers left-handed,
his right arm draped
over the top of the front seat.

I want to touch that blond-furred arm,
hold his fingers in my hand's hollow.

My mother leans to the right,
stares out the front window at the black asphalt
unwinding into the desert's lusterless gold.
She doesn't look at him or at me
or at the fifth of whiskey
amber-stilled next to her left foot.

Out the window to the left,
a mountain presses purple up up
until lead clouds block the ascension
and, through that metallic gray,
God shoots silver shafts just for me.

Give me the bottle, Edith,
he says to my mother.
I see the dip of her left shoulder,
hear the slap of the bottle against his hand.

Her gaze never leaves the ochre-scrubbed sand.

He tilts the Jim Beam—
the scorched yellow liquid flows
into his mouth. I hear him gulp and swallow.
I see his fingers tender-curled
around the bottle's neck.

In the mirror, his crow's feet gentle
and his dishwater eyes flash
a moment's burnished blue—
not for my mother not for me not for himself
not for the saffron sand or the purple mountain
but for the brown-gold whiskey.

Out the window,
still purple, the mountain—
the white-gold slashing the stubborn gray,
not god-painted or angel-mounted—
a trick of the atmosphere, a sleight of the hand.

Jack of Hearts

Oh lord Disney, I kneel
before your reels of revelation in
     Sleeping Beauty.
I will follow the dogma and
sleep

              and sleep
      until...

Not even yellow-gold whiskey
surging at flood stage

           (is my mother drowning in
           my father's river)?
will wake me.

When the prince, astride an ornate
dragon flashing sequined scales,
swoops through my open window,
he will kiss my barely breathing mouth.

I will jail words of dissent,

           (my father isn't a real prince,
           how can you be?)
no matter how hard they catapult
against clenched teeth,
the white-minted gate stays shut.

Tall, wavy blond hair, lake-blue eyes, he will have
a crooked smile

           (he reminds of someone,
           another prince,
           a not-real-prince)
we will ride away he will hold me so close we will seem as

     one.

My mouth unlocks,
all the do-not-believe-in-him words
will tumble out, splatter the purple sky with
      small
      angry
      black bits
      of chaos.

I will ask the prince,
as we streak through the crystal-studded void,
can I sleep on a goose-down bed
littered with blue satin pillows?
Will you clutter my naked body
with hundreds of jewels? And
will you give me a heart beating

                        red silk?

In a voice, mining silver depths,
he says, *I am your prince, your savior.*
With your pink shell-shaped hand
scoop out your heart.
Offer it to me.
I will snatch it and cram it into my mouth.
Do not be concerned. In your empty chest cavity
    I will left-center my heart.
        No, not beating silk.
          Not even red.

Burn White

Amber whiskey sloshes
out of the chipped
white motel mug
as he chases down
down the white pills.
Dozens.
Of those little white pills.
He collapses on the white sheets,
body blanched white.
Like the scattered
unswallowed
pills.

My mother is sent for.
My mother drives to the motel.
My mother views the body.
Sprawled on the now not so
white sheets.
The blue washed
out of his eyes.
His body death-stilled.
His voice quieted to white noise
she will never stop hearing.

My Father, the Tree

My father is dead,
not gone. I know because
I see his upper body leaf-crowded,
his arms about to thin and divide into bent
and arching branches, torso soon to thicken and
lengthen into a steadfast trunk. Leaves caress his face
and emboss their pattern on his shrinking skin. His watered-
down blue eyes round with fear and sorrow and regret
for kissing death on the mouth. Before stained
glass green usurps his sight, before leaves
curl through his nose, before stems
spiral down his throat, his words
flutter like the wind
ruffling
leaves.
Will I be
able to keep
my heart? he asks
No, the tree god answers,
although you will spin rings throughout your being.

Down the Hatch

Somewhere someone shoots a gun inside his mouth
not my father he shot pills with a whiskey chaser down
his committed throat
I remember
he drank and drank until his face bloated his eyes washed
out his stomach protruded
I remember
he hit a policeman who then arrested him took him to jail
we bailed him out he went to a motel
I remember
the very next morning he called my mother said *goodbye*
I love you she said *I love you too*
I remember
the very next morning after that morning the motel
requested no begged my mother to
come not in ten minutes get here before the moment
spreads its stain
I remember
her words raced down the hall to the bathroom where I
was applying green eyeshadow
he's dead he's dead by his own hand that brought the
glass of whiskey to his mouth to
wash down dozens of pills that make you sleep forever if
you take enough
I remember
that I forgot what happened next.

Unsaid Sentences

Tattooed on the back of my eyelids
your smile crumpled
in the dregs of Jim Beam gold,
your eyes rinsed of color,
no longer the blue that once
caught me midair,
your body still
as the freezer ice waiting
for the whiskey melt,
your voice rusted out,
your words so ragged
they scrape my soft parts.

Why choose bourbon's pyrite love
over mine, are my said love
words not shiny enough?
What if I pry open my tarnished scratched
armor to free caged unsaid sentences?
Look daddy here is what I am not pretty enough
not smart enough not brave enough
and how can you give me life lessons
when you hug Johnnie Walker, listen
to his secrets not mine not,
my sisters' not
my mother's?

Why do we even let ourselves love?

You were the emperor of ice cream,
the king of coloring books, the mayor of praline
candies, the man who danced with my little feet
on your polished Florsheim plain-toe shoes,
who whirled me on to your lap
and sang

Trottie Horsie don't fall down
    And spill the baby's candy,
        you plunged me so close so close to the floor,
          at the very last moment swooped me up,
            both of us weightless with laughter.

You and Momma drank martinis before dinner
(maybe meat loaf and baked potatoes, my favorite).

Once my mother told me she wished she had not
drunk those martinis with him
or any other kind of drink.

I tasted the dregs of their Old Fashioneds.
So sweet, so caustic.

II. DARK

Gangsters of the Portland Sky

Everywhere they black-litter lawns,
stutter-hop on buckled sidewalks,
cake-walk down Willamette Boulevard,
and flutter-kick away from speeding cars'
smash and gash at the minute's last flicker.
They recognize faces, post sentries
in bare-branched trees, screech coded warnings—
beware of us, the gangsters of the Portland sky!
We dive bomb red-tail hawks mid thermal swirl
and catcall their retreating swoop.

I have often wondered
whether it is better to know
a little about a lot or a lot about a little.
I could google crows, learn more about them—
every day observe their black bird actions
and stop studying my own behavior,
stop trying to understand why blood pumps
red outside my body but looks blue in my veins
and why the beats of my heart slow
to an almost stillness when I think
of my father who lies in his grave
but is not dead.

I do know something that is not a poem
instead a naked fact.
Once I saw lying in a street island's center
a dead crow encircled by a small cadre of crows
and on some arcane signal
they all bowed.

Death Takes My Mother

On the strands of a spider web
the sun plucks
an overture of light.
The sky's blue vibrates
and a nearby rose sings
a lipstick-red aria—

the color my mother wore,
although when dying,
her unpainted mouth radiated
pink that I kissed over and over
whispering wake up wake up
please wake up.

Center-stilled
in a light-storm of symmetry,
a spider waits for a passerby
who, blinded by the threads' flash,
will dive headfirst into the sink
of those sinuous strands.

My mother sways and stumbles
into the web's silken stick—
no fight, not even a token scuffle,
as the spider, jaws agape,
scuttle-stops,
scuttle-stops
nearer and nearer.
I shut my eyes, lay my face
against the rose of her cheeks—
so close to her soul,
his fangs graze my heart.

Remains of My Mother

Very soon after she died, I had my mother cremated. We buried her dust-sized bone fragments next to my dad's body. Of course, his flesh was long gone—no dust either, all kinds of things devour the corpse not just maggots. When I last saw my mother, pink grazed her cheeks, her once straight hair now white-whorled against her neck, no death rattle just a faint buzz, her breath cinnamon-scented. I know because I kissed her lips, not cold and ashy, her face not white with her absence. She wasn't dead yet. Once my mother and I sat across each other at the kitchen table drinking coffee, waiting for the whole day to live through. My father called from the motel where he spent the night after we bailed him out for assaulting a police officer we called because he violated the restraining order. He phoned her to say goodbye. I am not talking about for the day. For the week. For the month. For the year. For the decade. But for the rest of his life, for the rest of our lives. I think he said *I love you* because she said *I love you too* and then hung up.

Shades of White

Rollo has moved, the most beloved dog on Yale Street, a white Siberian Husky, also the most beautiful. With eyes the color of a calving glacier and his coat not the white of skim milk, instead cream flecked with gold. His mouth is soft, he takes my proffered treat with velvet gentleness. His coat is soft, my fingers sink into creamy depths. He is the exemplar of white, better than the clouds rounding and ballooning in the sky's blue zenith, better than the magnolias which aren't really white, instead pale ivory, and the flowers my mother spray-painted gold to wind through the banister at Christmas. Her hair was not white then nor were her small hands. Her left-hand fingers were damaged in a car accident when she was young yet a hand just the right size for holding mine, even as adults. To hide the bent fingernails, she painted them with the *Love That Red* nail polish. Always. She hated her light brown hair too fine, too straight. As she lay dying, her hair the color of Rollo's curled around her neck but she didn't know it, she was in a coma. After she died, I suspect her hands turned white. I refused to view the body.

The Dark Inside Light

When snow splinters the winter light
into millions of micro suns,
no white is whiter.

Not the stars' sequined sprinkle
nor wind-scudded clouds
nor the foam floating on the wave's edge.

When crows crackle their black
and shatter the white silence,
no black is blacker.

Not rain-slicked slate
nor a moon-absent night
nor coal glittering on hidden rock walls.

When we die, does the blackest of black
roll over us until we disappear
into a Vantablack abyss

or do we disintegrate into thousands
and thousands of ions the sun scintillates
in the snow stretched over the lawn?

White seems a better way to go
until I think of my mother's hands—
when dead, the whitest of all.

Her Eyelids Like Autumn Leaves

Forever sadness
storms her eyes
after he dies,
her husband, my father.
Those eyes remember him
at the motel.
Dead,
not of natural causes.
Pain burrs her voice
when she speaks to me.
She thinks she did not love
us enough,
him enough.
He is the one
who did not love enough.
He sloughed his body,
pushed his heart
through a membrane thinner
than the skin of her eyelids
where love is blind,
love is deadlocked.

Before she left her body,
her skin turned
gold and thin
like an autumn leaf
about to float
down or away or somewhere,
maybe where she is now,
where I want to be
if only the autumn sun
would burn my skin gold.

My Mother's Molecules

My mother's diamond floats
on a gold chain circling my neck.
No use licking the hard-faceted surface.
The rub of her everyday life, the caress
of my throat's hollow
have long worn off her molecules.

Inside—
a scattering of my mother's molecules
has seeped through to the core
where they hide in the tiny flaws
within this V2-rated diamond.
I fractal myself small enough
to squeeze into one of those
microscopic inclusions
and nestle my scintilla
next to my mother's. A chemical reaction

(could it be love?)

unites our molecules and

no need
for words, the snowflakes
of communication, mere flickers
of gleam that evaporate before your eye
can register the white glint.
Instead, her gem-captured essence flows
through my compressed iota.

I am nine.

Again.

Into the kitchen
yellow-warmed, oven-warmed,
first hot day of the year warmed,
redolent with baking apple pie,
my sister and I scamper.
My mother places into our greedy hands
our favorite treat, fresh
out-of-the-oven-rolled piecrust,
cinnamon, sugar and butter layered.
Mouth filled with the flakey treat, I beg,
Can we go barefoot?
Can we run through the sprinklers?
Please, please?

We scramble outside.
The sky burns blue,
the jade-tinted grass tickles
the arches of our feet, squirms
through our toes. Squealing,
we run through the water's
rainbow curve, weave
through the six hard-spraying fountains,
squawk when the cold slaps
our pink-white child-smooth skin,
shriek when our dad chases
us with the hose and spritzes us—
each droplet encapsulating
my father's grin, my sister's dimpled smile.
Their eyes are the sky that grips the sun.

We are giggled-stuffed
until our laughter escapes
like air hissing out of a balloon. We laugh
and laugh and until lighter than air,
to the top of the sky we drift,
break through the navy-blue ribbon

into black ruffled silk.
We are floating diamonds,
out-glittering
the nearby starshine.

Sutton Hoo

i.
The people lay his body
their king, their savior, in his ship
not to be sea-launched,
the people know the ocean's power
to grind   to pound   to smash   to flay
his proud vessel   to boil
away every drop of his sacred body.
He would be no more
before the sea wound
around the globe.

The people's love looms larger
than the ocean's stretch across the horizon.
Their love staggers their hearts
impels their hands   their arms   their legs
to pull   to drag   to heave
the ship inland where they
dig   and   gouge   and   scoop
out yards and yards of soil
to create a cavern whose sides and bottom
embrace his ship,
the ship that shelters his beloved body,
the ship whose arms hold his myriad treasures—
a gold shoulder clasp inlaid with garnets and glass
ten silver bowls
a ceremonial helmet
a shield
a sword
a lyre
a silver plate from the Byzantine Empire.

In this sanctified cavity
they pile   they pack   they carry   they cram

enough earth to make a hillock
for those love-driven enough to visit
on the hallowed grave

                          and weep.

Almost a millennium passes.
A man who loves
                all loved things buried

shovels aside yards and yards and yards
of soil and there lies
              the ship
                  still breathing
                        love.

See the ribs, the keel stamped into the mire.
See the cradling soil, the protecting earth.
See the treasures the massive love
holds in thrall.

ii.
What if I excavate my father, my once
but not future king?
When I scoop out the lungs
crack open the ribs—
no valentine shape throbs
with life's carmine mysteries,
instead, a chaotic organ, soldier-chewed.
Did he wear it on his sleeve
or perhaps pin it on the left side
    of his Navy-issued shirt?
See the soldiers—the ones dying of homesickness,
terror, and especially those who lean toward
the black, thick with mystery—
tear off   bite off   slice off

slabs   hunks   chunks   bits
until what is left
                        is not.

What if I excavate my mother? Easy
to bend open the smooth satin ribs.
Left centered, a heart ruffled and tiered
like a rose, silken, crimson
I long to caress.
First, I must grasp the thorned stem,
(the backbone sorrow-cracked, pain-splintered),
yes, it punctures my too-soft hand
but I must not let go—
her husband-memories merge
with my father-memories.
See his true love, alcohol, drown his love
for her   for me   for my sisters
see him scrabble into his grave
                        before he is dead
I see   I see   I see.

Now I can settle my heart next to hers
both of us unfold   unfold   unfold
our tightly wound petals until
our yellow gold-feathered centers
whisper our treasure.

III. LOVE

The Weight of Grief

An apple center-rests in my hand,
green-yellow satin caresses the skin,
my mouth waters for the tart crunch,
the sweet syrup.

Stop! The wolf, tethered
behind my heart, whisper-growls,

Apples are earth-bound.
Taste the moon instead.

I glance at my palm.
There downsized to fit
into my hand's heart,
a luminous sphere.
The surface rocks and bumps
against my skin, the yellow hue
not apple-shined but glimmer-glistened.

I bite into the icy globe,
my body billows cool,
and my weight dwindles.

I press my hand against my thinning skin,
ask the wolf, *if I lick*
the golden shimmer dripping
through my fingers,
will I lift off?
I long to float up—
or need I take another bite?

Through clenched teeth
the wolf hisses,

Static grief weighs you down.
You still mourn your mother
although her ashes, littered
with bone fragments, have nestled
next to your father's casket for 15 years.
You kill your father
over and over
although 50 years
have stripped his flesh
from his bones.
Can you not see
how they shine in his tomb?

Eat the whole thing.

Then will I round, exude white-gold,
slide up the purple-suede sky
telescope-spotted
as a perfect moon miniature,
waxing joy?

Yes, and so hallowed
from your meteoric rise,
at the next high mass
the moon will swallow your being.

Moon Mad

A pumped-up moon breaks
through my bedroom window
sheets me with ivory satin.
Listen to me, his dark-side voice
growls in my right ear,
I rough up my blankness with black lace
gorge on shine and graze women's
empty thighs with white silk.
The bored-black sky thrills
when my coin face hard-kisses the horizon
and what do I get?
A lone wolf's grief-spattered howl.

He presses lips icy-hot against my cheek,
his man-in-the-moon eyes whisper
Come on baby, sing me sacred
I will gild your skin white-gold.
Kneel to me.
I will surge your salt,
tsunami wave your blood,
smooth your jagged,
cream your dark.

My left eye beams my answer.
This body's too slight a vessel
for all that white-hot.
I'll blow up, shoot out dwarf stars.
But if you float up to the up
and size down to a communion wafer
I will open my mouth,
you can slip down my throat,
shine holy in my new-moon void.

White with Absence

Thud. A hummingbird mistakes the sliding glass door for air. Falls to the welcome mat. On his side, he lies still as the white painted on the morning sky. He's dead, he must be dead. My hand scoops up a being lighter than the whoosh of my breath. So in love with this tiny perfection, I begin to squeeze, but if he isn't really dead, a crush born of passion will kill him. It's hard to stop, I have to stop. Bob squeezed. He necklaced my throat with purple fingerprints that sank down and down through my flesh, through my muscles, through my bones, enlarging, expanding until my whole body received their message that love does not fly with the wings of a white dove. He stopped before he killed me. For several weeks I wore his gift—a choker of purple-blue symmetrical smudges on my pale, almost white skin. The hummingbird's eye flashes open, he startles in my hand's palm, flits away on wings whirring a thousand times a minute. Traffic signal red iridescence flares from his throat. Almost lethal, such honed beauty. In my hand a white absence.

Her Hair So White

When I last saw my mother alive her once straight hair
    white-whorled,
pink grazed her cheeks she breathed out cinnamon and
    sighed *goodbye.*

I kissed her lips not cold her face not white with her
    absence,
no death rattle just a faint buzz sliding into goodbye.

When you die your blood drains to the bottom of your
    body.
I refused to view my mother's dead-white face and kiss her
    goodbye.

Next to my dad her boxed dust-body lies forever stilled,
his body devoured by maggots and things to feed the
    goodbye.

Once my dad battered his way through the restraining
    order,
pushed the policeman then smashed his face with a right
    hook goodbye.

In the morning my mother and I sat drinking black coffee,
the night before we bailed out my father and cried out
    goodbye.

In the morning the telephone rang he craved goodbye,
not for a night nor a month, a forever goodbye.

My mother said I love you too and not one word more,
hung up on a world of love forever and honeyed goodbyes.

I am still alive I cannot abide the word goodbye,
I am still alive sometimes I pray for a splintered goodbye.

Walking Point

My husband walks on the cusp of his focus,
allows his gaze a five-yard sweep.
When he sees a spider web glint
in the fierce green monotony,
his left leg starts a forward motion.
His right foot digs into the mud
as his gaze traces the shining thread
to the ground.
Not spider-made.
A wire strand burrowed into the soil.
He walks point for his squad.

Watch the high curb,
my husband warns me
while we walk on a downtown sidewalk.
He pulls me away from a passing car's
arcing spray. At home, I search
the black-clouded abyss for the dead
arms of my mother stretching
open to embrace me. I teeter
on the edge. My husband holds me back.
He walks point for me.

An angel lives inside my husband,
a savage angel whose wings encircle
the softest section of his core.
For his hospice patients
only a wind's hush of tenderness escapes.
Just a thin piece of my love can slant
in between the sharp-edged platinum feathers.
He walks point for his heart.

The Moon Knows I Am in Love

erratic oval
elongated bloated
pasted in see-through
not quite navy-blue air
eye-level moon
way too big
for the immature sky

not stark white this moon
gold-smoothed
no not smooth
moony holes patched
with ragged blotches

lunatic moon
slides over to the driver's
right side
then to the left
then can't be seen
soon coffee-cream
magnet moon adheres
to the windshield

man in the moon
laughs and laughs
offers me a drink
I sip the missing edge
both of us are sliding
off the sky I am drunk
my body shines moonbeams
that slither through the sky
and streak the asphalt

I swallow
the moon whole
my body stretches
and stretches until the skin
glides open
my heart floats out
a new Moon

Love Meditation

Come sit next to me,
my husband invites.
Breathe in the morning's white air.
Watch your breath curl red
down your throat, swirl aquamarine
on the way out.

My eyes skitter,
my attention swerves.
Nothing
in nature meditates, I whisper.

Yes, he says, *trees, they breathe*
in soot-laden air, breathe
out green-golden truth.

I elongate my body into a two branched tree.
I inhale my husband's essence, exhale
rainbow shimmer.

If one day his breathing stutters
to a stop and he topples
to the ground—an unearthed maple tree—
without his shade,
the sun will set fire to my leaves,
my branches, my trunk, even my roots.

My Husband Loves Winter

Clean, he says, *and clear.*
Look into the heart of the forest,
the angle of the tree bones—sharp, crooked, naked.
Sometimes the winter sun spreads
pale gold between charcoal-hued alders,
see the air beneath the hawk's wings
and in the shadows, the flash
of a coyote's eyes?

He can still his vision, quiet his heart,
and study the scattered twigs,
the squirrel's pelt—the divination,
he declares, to life's mystery.

When a rainbow arcs across a lead-heavy sky,
he looks not at the swoop
of primary colors
but at the sharp-edged trees inked
on the austere horizon.

Beautiful, he says.

The Real Factual Bird

Shubunkin goldfish flash cobalt, green, crimson,
and charcoal gray in the two adjoining backyard ponds.
My husband loves them, watches over them, counts
the babies darting glimmers of nascent colors.

He places a life-sized blue heron statue at the end of
the lower pond to stop the real herons from swooping down
for an appetizer.

But racoons scoop up bitefulls after bitefulls until
the shubunkins are no more.
My husband bows his head, his eyes blue-glitter with tears.

Now the peeling faded statue stands guard over empty
gold-brown water.

This morning, three feet away from the sliding-glass doors
stands the statue.
Did my husband move him?

No, not a figure—the real factual bird,
sleekly motionless, a foot taller than the statue.

His light-filled body looms the gray of the first morning
light and the white of cotton sheets billowing on
the clothes line. His wings suddenly unfurl and spread out
and out and out. He waves them three times to reach the
cumulous cloud's stormy edge.

Flow the Ending Letter

Magenta—
my mind careens
searching for an image of that hue.
Maybe pink on steroids
or red having sex with ultramarine.
If words were containers
filled with what they mean,
when I say—magenta—
fuchsia would explode out of my mouth.
If write it, I can just graze the meaning,
not with a scanty scrawl
but with calligraphic pen strokes—
bold lines, graceful swirls—
although not enough to corral
more than a quick glance.
Eyes want color, gleam and glimmer.
I choose my favorite nib,
mix water, gum arabic,
red-pink pearlescent powder,
dip a small paint brush into the shiny liquid,
stroke a dab into the nib's concavity.
With agonizing care, I press the pen
down on cold-press watercolor paper—
surface rough enough to form
tiny hills and valleys
throughout the line's straight stretch—
let up the pressure,
then at the end of the stroke
push down again so that
both the beginning
and the end swell slightly.
Then I twirl the descenders,
flow the ending letter.

I need to begin and end the day
as tender and mindful—
press down
on the sight of my husband's
good morning smile,
curl up against my dachshund's
clever body at night,
stretch my life out
in a straight magenta
not quite smooth line.

Old Love

My husband writes me love notes
on the shells of hardboiled eggs.
His eyes are underwater blue.
When he listens, his body stills
like a blade of grass
in a windless lawn.
He tells me young love
is a bludgeoning waterfall
but old love drips on a craggy boulder,
shapes the roundness into unending.

IV. MOON

The Crow and I Have a Conversation

Poet

My husband tosses stale hamburger buns topped with sesame seeds on the grass, sometimes leaves the garbage lid ajar. For you. I write poems about you; how you outwit falcons, spit in the face of motorized danger, strut like a majordomo dressed in black satin. I am crazy about your conventions on telephone wires even though you argue for hours. I wish I knew about what. I understand your love of bling. I collect sparkly things too. If I could cradle you in my hand, I would stroke those silk feathers and kiss your clever beak. Maybe in the center of my palm, your feet would scratch out a love message to me.

Crow

Every morning I shine my black-feathered tuxedo, hone my beak and sharpen my eyes to the snapping point. If you tried to hold me, I would bite your fingers, claw warnings in your palm. I make tools to access the narrowest difficulty. I hide sparklies where you will never find them. I am dangerous. I sometimes fly solo but when falcons veer into my airspace, my gang has by back. Crows do not argue on telephone wires; they catch up on the day's events like how my daughter just missed the jaws of a motor-monster or my sister is teaching her babies to fly. Sometimes we discuss you or other two-trunked barkless trees, how ugly you are with only two leafless limbs. No wonder you cover them with pieces of colored cloth. Of course, you write poems about us. Who wouldn't? We are wild, we are beautiful. We fly, we soar, we float, we strut our ebony-breasted stuff. In the evening we gather in murders, lock wings and sing a paean for our dead. We breathe out dark smoke as we sleep. We are the reason night is black.

Giant Pacific Octopus at the Hatfield Marine Science Center

I wait.

                So long I have been waiting.

For a land-being to free me
from this caged aloneness.
Little do I care that they are sizeable tubes,
        lumpy
          with two
        uncurved stalk-
        like arms stuck
         to her sides
         and two for
     standing on   the outside
of this seawater-filled, hard-air barriered,
see-through prison.

Not like me,
with eight arms to
    curl
        swirl
            spiral
        curve
   arc.

You land-beings on the other side of the barrier
with those bulbous white, blue or brown
circle-centered eyes,
can see my majesty.
Yes, you,
who spread your fibrous fingers
on the surface where I splay my body.
What do you want?
        Not that I care.

Indifference stains my body pale.

I wait.
                    Then.
                         Above me!
                                  In a flesh-colored
                                                    flash

                         she appears.
She is unlike the other tubes.
She sees who I am.

I blaze crimson, unfurl two
of my arms to shoot out of the water,
bracelet
her
   wrists
          (without squeezing),
stroke the shelled crab she offers,
fold it in my second arm's efficient circle,
place it in my mouth politely, never greedily.

She tosses me colored balls.
The big yellow one, my favorite, I loop
into my sixth arm. My eighth arm
curls around the red ball and swishes
it toward my mouth's opening.
An octopus joke,
I won't eat it.

I long to wind
all eight arms around her torso,
pull her in to be my playmate, my friend
for
all of
the time.

No, what I really want—
to envelope her in my arms' soft spiral
until after dark. We can escape
to the boundaryless ocean.
I will protect her.
From orcas, sharks, Moray eels.
Anything, everything.
I will squirt a black ink curtain
to hide her, or cover
her body with mine,
quick-changed
to look like a sea-boulder.

I know, I know, she cannot breathe the seawater.
And, although
I might be able to drag myself out,
the hard air stutters and slices
through my gills
and I slide-stick
on the unyielding surface.

You might not know this.
I have three
hearts.
Necessary to pump copper-rich blood
to my
supple
muscular arms.

Three hearts that can break.

Indifferent Moon

The siren's red orange sound pushes through the stony air, a buzzsaw whine slicing molecules into quarks that stipple the atmosphere. Sometimes dogs answer with a deep-throated gold satin aria, and the moon wishes it were night so she could paint her answer with milky shine. She loves dogs and wolves and foxes and lovers and all who gaze with adoration into her deep-set eyes, not that she cares about our little sufferings like how my husband feels, how I feel when he mislays words. Often. He searches, I search but they are weightless, colorless, odorless. He grasps at them only to open his hand and find darting molecules and quarks, no words. They litter the floor. I scoop them up, open my hand, show him. *No*, he says, *not the ones I wanted*. I roll them around until they center-bunch in my hand's palm, slide them off to lob at the moon. No use singing them to her, she has no ears. Neither does the sun, who speaks to no one except sunflowers who smolder their welcome, see flames shoot out the circumference of their burnt sienna centers.

Eyebrow Bear

Every night my husband sleeps
with Eyebrow Bear,
a teddy he rescued, mud-caked,
tossed to the curb, but intact,
a baby proof bear with black stitched eyes
and high-arched brown yarn eyebrows.
A bear so soft and bendable,
the washing machine cannot not rip
or even ruffle him.

Eyebrow bear knows inside my husband—
no cotton stuffing—
instead tumbling gems of love.
He doesn't care
my husband loses words.
Where do they all go? On the floor
next to where my husband sits,
stands or sleeps? Do they swim
in an unknown pond treading
water until he rescues them?

Why do we even let ourselves love?
Eyebrow Bear will not die,
but my husband will.
In the meantime, I am losing
him inch by inch—
death in slow motion.
And I can't hold him fast.

The Poet and the Dragon

The Poet caresses the dragon's gilded scales, breathes out words of love. Not a full-frontal declaration—feather-flames sometimes whoosh out his careless mouth, crisscross scars on the Poet's left forearm. No matter, he dotes on the dragon's golden lamella, scarlet spikes, purple eyes. He even sleeps on the floor next to his bed where the dragon curls his sinuous length into three glittering coils.

The poet pleads, *breathe into my mouth, enough heat and warm my words to forty-nine degrees Celsius. My audience will burn without blistering.*

The dragon answers, a flicker of fire escapes his red-hued fanged mouth. *First you have to feed me.*

I have nothing but my fealty to offer, the poet answers while flexing his empty fingers.

The dragon's amethyst gaze floods the poet's eyes. *Nice but not enough. I want what you love. I want your mother. I want your lover. I want your children. I want your brother.*

The dragon snorts black smoke threaded with scarlet scintillas—carbonized mist the Poet inhales. Instantaneously his fingers twine a pen. Out pour words so hot with meaning they will scald fingers, scorch eyes, sear hearts.

Still with him. His children. His mother. His brother.

But the dragon eats his lover.

    ***

Two tattooed
big-eyed
Chinese dragons
scaled in rainbow colors,
wind up my husband's body.
Their heads rest over his shoulders,
eyes fix on his heart.
Their goal—
block
bite
burn
soot-black
word-eating
beasts.

The dragons tire.
Dozens
of word-starved monsters
find their way
into my husband's mouth,
rappel down his throat,
settle in his word cache
where they rip
and tear
and gobble
entire sentences,
whole paragraphs.
But not the word *love*,
clutched
in my husband's left hand.

Deep Sea Fishing

Over and over
my husband and I fish
for words swimming in his inner
white-capped darkening sea.
He pulls back his rod,
casts the line, reels in, throws again.

                      Nothing.

Through gritted teeth he says,
the fish aren't biting.
I teeter on the edge of the boat
Please, please don't

                      give up.

He stays his arm on the upswing,
stares at the unyielding gray.
I saw it on the news, he mutters.
They advance toward …
The Russians? I ask.
Yes, we have one of the …
up the Columbia River … a power … a
…

Power plant? I try to picture what he means—
A transfer station? Here in Portland?
    No, No, No! in Washington. He snaps the pole,
I cast my line. *Do you mean*
the nuclear power station in the Tri Cities?
A large fish arcs out of the water.
Yes, he says.
The fish takes the bait.
I yank the word out of the clinging ocean,

                      net it.

We lay it on the table—

a sinewy strong word, it twists and contorts.
Both of us grasp it, use all our strength
to pin it down.

Chernobyl.

The fish are learning how to elude us,
populating in his ocean-drenched interior
deeper and deeper they go.
Are they not part of his self?
The true essential self that makes him

Himself?

Superman, Can You Help?

Ok Superman, where are you? Speeding faster than the hurtling wind about to tear up the Atlantic Coast? Aiming for the blue center of the hurricane, one of God's many eyes? You won't find the meaning of life in that silent crush of massive indifference but stay suspended in that sapphire's slow pulse—a place you can take a break from all that begging. How many trains can you right? How many bombs can you batter? And what about the countless bullet barrages, the thousands and thousands that thunk against your steely chest, and no one says thank you. Instead fusillades of rage-amped pleas pummel you— *hold back global warning! Kapow the virus's ravaging army! Swallow the oncoming cyclone! Slam shut the earthquake's crashing chasm!* No wonder you ponder a place in one of God's eyes. Listen, Superman. I am drowning and I need saving. Yes, I know, I know, I am just one person's voice in the seethe of barbed words stalking that shell-shaped ear. Please, please let all those suffering-soaked words swim through your ear canal—down, down until they strike your aorta's eyes. Can you help my husband? He can't speak most words. Sometimes we grab one of the fish flashing through the heaving sentences, clutch tight before they pop out so we can examine the iridescence for meaning. Slippery too slippery. Please, Superman, help me cradle his words, not squeeze.

Sterling

My husband doesn't like tea.
Neither do I.
I can't say
           how about a cuppa?
We drink coffee,
a wake-up get-through-another day drink,
not like tea—an all-day-anytime drink,
a reason to relax into a long chat
with a cup of strong sweetened Earl Grey
with a dash of milk, no lemon
except we don't drink tea
and he never chats.
How could he?
Hundreds of his words
can't find his mouth.
They drown deep
they drown dark
in his Mariana Trench.

I have friends,
four friends
who know what I don't know,
how strenuous, how arduous, how deep, how often
I dive.
They say we *understand,*

        this is
        so
        hard
        for
        you.

I plan a tea party just for them.
Earl Grey tea steeps in the gilded blue teapot.
On my mother's Candlewick Clear platters
coconut-flavored layer cake, buttercream frosted,
and caramel-slicked chocolate brownies,
crustless sandwiches—buttered radish,
curried egg salad, goat cheese with olives—
served on my mother's fluted rose pattern plates
set between my good flatware
(not sterling like my mother's,
like she was).
My husband stops by the ivory lace-draped table
where a Lennox vase blooms tulips
egg yolk yellow, lipstick red.
He smiles at my friends' furrowed faces,
softly mounded stomachs, sloping bosoms,
silver-stranded hair.
When some of his words
(oh such wanted words),
won't rise to the surface,
each one of the four friends (more sterling
than my mother's ornate silverware)
jump in his ocean, and each one
surfaces with just the right word—
not even out of breath.

A Star, Not a Skeleton

My husband has a kind of dementia. His brain pitches out words before he can catch them and hand them to me. Time and time again. No use combing the air, they dissolve into meaningless mist. He can no longer move his body in a smooth coordinated way. When he falls, the ground heaves and buckles until I fall too. Not on the floor but into a space between dead and alive where monsters wait to tear off pieces of my heart and eat them. *Are you all right?* I bleat, *please be all right.* Once he fell backward down two stairs. He cracked his head open. He was all right. Emergency room all right. MRI all right. Ten stitches all right. He will probably die before I do. The other night he fell asleep in front of the TV. Half of his open mouth slid over to the side. I shouted, *Ron, Ron!* But he didn't move. I wanted to grab death around the neck and kill it. Then he woke up. After he dies, I will find a gun. I will point it at the mortician and order him, *peel off his skin. Tear off his musculature. Give me the skeleton. Now, right now.* I will carry his bones in my fleshed-out arms, settle him in the seat next to me and drive home. At least once I will turn to him, smile fondly and say *I love you.* I will paint his skull ribs arms legs feet everything gold. I will place my mother's diamond in one eye socket and the aquamarine ring he gave me in the other. On creamy silk sheets, I will position his frame on its side. I will lie down and place his skeleton arms around me, and he will say *I don't reside in my bones. Those jewels are not my eyes. Look at the ribcage, do you see a heart? I am gone away far away. I am a star not a bright supergiant but a red dwarf your naked eye will never be able to see even in the Mohave Desert, but I am there. Waiting.*

V. SKY

The Hereafter

I am nearing the dark.
Gathered in tight murders,
crows watch
and bow
to the ink-stained cloud
closing in on me.

The sun casts a sidelong glance
then drops
to the other side of the world,
too bored
with the dark,
too bored
with me
to watch the gloom advancing.

As the coal-dark shadow approaches
nearby stars
watch,
pulse,
and scatter glitter
coating my body in star-shed.

An angel spies my gleaming body—
not a sculpted angel
waving creamy wings,
an angel darker
than a black hole
folds me
into his stormy plumage,
flies me
to the star of his choice,

and flings me
into a flare erupting from the corona.

Beside me my mother flames.

I Cannot Kiss the Sky

Evening.

Light scattered in the gloaming
reveals houses etched
black, the sky flooded
in luminous indigo,
a sky that holds my mother,
her memory.
No that's not it.
She is the sky,
that shimmering purple-blue.
I cannot kiss it,
I cannot gather it in my arms,
I cannot even touch it.

Morning.

Facing the bathroom mirror,
in honor of her
I apply mascara, hot-curl my hair.
Always, she fixed her hair,
never wore housecoats,
painted her fingernails
Love That Red,
her lips too. That lipstick
could not hide
that slight tremor when her wide mouth
smiled nor distract
from the sadness saturating her gray eyes.

The shape of my face
echoes hers
but not my unlipsticked thin lips
pursed into a moue of sorrow

nor my light eyes,
although grief prowls behind
the blue-green façade.

Come back, Momma,
please comeback.
Curl your hand with the accident-damaged
fingers into mine,
press your soft barely fuzzed
check next to mine.
Call me *dear*.
I exert all the love inside of me,
Come back, Momma.
I am waiting.

Apple of Perfect Love

My mother peels white-green,
tart-sweet pippins
until yellow-green ribbons coil
on the counter, decorate the linoleum floor.
Each strip unbroken.

Her piecrust, almost transparent, she places
with unprecedented tenderness
atop the apple slices piled high
on the welcoming bottom crust.
How does she roll out both sheets
into diaphanous layers?

How does she marry the tissue-paper thin dough
to the glass pie plate
without shreds separating and
smudging the kitchen floor?

I am not making apple pie.
Pie crust eludes me.
Pieces stick to the rolling pin,
smear the cutting board.
Swear words float through the fog of flour.

However, I am peeling apples.
No matter how often,
how strenuously,
I order my hands to skin
each apple
                in one continuous crimson sheet,
strips stutter and spike on the tiles.

I stopped trying to recreate her apple pies.
I stopped searching bakeries, restaurants, dinner parties

for perfection's pinnacle—
love-grazed pippins,
wed to cinnamon, sugar, butter, lemon,
almost friable crust tender-blanketing
the apples, vanilla ice cream melting
on a V-shaped piece placed
on her fluted rose-patterned China.

Instead, I make apple cake,
sassy with Fuji chunks,
replete with cinnamon, brown sugar, butter,
moist to the point of crumbliness,
but not
                  perfect.

Fundamental Forces of the Universe

Unseen, cached beyond the night sky,
science-ignored, exists the fifth fundamental

force: *love*—although not as strong
as the electromagnetic force but stronger

than gravity. A velvet hammer
that assaults my inner and outer body

at four o'clock in the morning. It hurts
my skin, my fat, the gray bones gleaming

in the dark of my body where it lives—
not in my veins, aorta, skeleton, muscles

not even in my heart but in whatever
clutches it white-knuckled

tight. I don't know who knows
if love even exists in the realm

of the real earth, the true universe.
Perhaps a chimerical hallucination

yet so corporeal, a glittering
sugar mountain glutting my made-up

heart not the real heart
although it thuds with an echoing

pain when I think of my mother,
I think of her all the time, her gray

sad-soaked eyes, her accident-damaged
left hand resting in my love-famished right.

The Weight of Soft

Cold-shredded clouds
down-drift in silken motion.
Almost weightless, each speck's
sparkle-feather touch.

And yet—

powdery glitter masses on trees
until the weight of soft bends
and breaks branches
too big to imagine.

The frozen silence explodes.

All that white—
the street is white
the sky is white
my heart is white.

I could rest my head on a white mound,
let my body sink into a snow shroud
my last breath in—

white-fractured stars.

Notes

"The Dark Inside the Light"
Vantablack: a coating so black that spectrometers can't measure it.

"Sutton Hoo"
Sutton Hoo is the site of two early medieval cemeteries in Suffolk, England where a self-taught archaeologist unearthed an Anglo-Saxon burial ship dating from the 6th to 7th centuries.

"Walking Point"
In combat, the soldier who takes point; the soldier who assumes the first and most exposed position in a combat military formation; the lead soldier/unit advancing through hostile or unsecured territory.

"Giant Octopus at the Hatfield Marine Science Center"
The Giant Pacific Octopus is known to be rather shy and usually friendly towards humans, rarely using its dangerous features to inflict harm.
            —from americanoceans.org › facts › giant-
                pacific-octopus

"The Five Fundamental Forces"
The four fundamental forces are:

Gravity, *the attraction between two objects that have mass or energy, turns out to be the weakest of the fundamental forces, especially at the molecular and atomic scales*

The weak force, *also called the weak nuclear interaction, is responsible for particle decay.*

The electromagnetic force *acts between charged particles,
like negatively charged electrons and positively charged
protons.*

The strong nuclear force *is the strongest of the four
fundamental forces. It's 6 thousand trillion trillion trillion
times stronger than the force of gravity, And that's because
it binds the fundamental particles of matter.*
        —from space.com

Acknowledgments

The author thanks and acknowledges the following publication where poems in this collection previously appeared, sometimes in alternate versions.

Autumn Voices: "Her Eyelids Like Autumn Leaves"

Bacopa Literary Review: "The Dark Inside the Light"

Central Oregon Writers Guild: "Eyebrow Bear"

Dove Tales: "Without a Life Vest"

Haunted Waters Press: "The Crow and I Have a Conservation"

Nostalgia Press: "Old Love"

Oprelle Newsletter: "Down the Hatch"

The Oregonian: "Gangsters of the Portland Sky"

Phantom Drift: "Death Takes My Mother," "The Hereafter"

She Holds the Face of the World (10th Anniversary Best of *Voicecatcher* Anthology): "The Hand-Off"

Voicecatcher: "The Hand-Off "

Website for Ageless Authors: "Gangsters of the Portland Sky," "The Moon Knows I'm in Love"

Whimsical Poet: "A is for Apple"

Poems included from my chapbook, *The Color of Goodbye*, published by Kelsay Books, 2021:
"Devil Doll"
"Without a Live Vest"
"The Hand-Off"
"My Father, the Tree"
"Death Takes My Mother"
"Her Eyelids Like Autumn Leaves"

Gratitude

I am deeply grateful to my sister, Kate MacMillan, for her loving and nonwavering support and encouragement.

I wrote most of these poems in classes taught by the inestimable Matthew Dickman. I owe him heartfelt thanks for his expert teaching, deep knowledge, keen wisdom, and incomparable kindness.

Thank you, dear MK Moen, for reading and commenting on every poem I write. Your generous support has helped me more than you know.

My deepest gratitude to Lana Hechtman Ayers for her belief in me and my work.

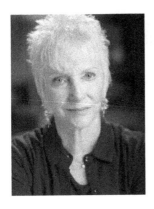

About the Author

An artist and poet, Pattie Palmer-Baker creates collages of her poetry using calligraphy and paste paper. Paste paper is an ancient decorative technique where paints are mixed with specially made paste on wet paper. Pattie creates and then cuts specific shapes and images to illustrate her poems written around the edges of the artwork. Her calligraphy is based on the 8th-century Carolingian letterforms established by Charlemagne in the latter part of the 8th and early 9th centuries.

The inspiration for and the meaning of the artwork always lies within the poem.

Over the years of exhibiting her artwork, she was surprised and delighted that people, despite what they may believe, do like poetry, and, in fact, many liked her poems more than the visual art. She now focuses solely on writing.

Nominated for the Pushcart Poetry Prize, and published in many journals including, *Poeming*

Pigeons Anthologies; Voicecatcher; The Best of Voicecatcher; Bacopa Literary Review, Military Experience & the Arts; Ghazal Page; Voices, The Art and Science of Psychotherapy; Calyx; and *Phantom Drift.* Palmer-Baker's work has received many awards, including First prize in the 2016 *Timberline Review,* First, Second, and the Bivona prize (for the best overall entry) in *Ageless Authors Anthology* 2019, First Prize in 2020 in the Central Oregon Writers' Guild contest, and First prize in the 2022 *Oprelle Oxbow* contest. Her chapbook, *The Color of Goodbye,* was recently published by Kelsay Books.

CPSIA information can be obtained
at www.ICGtesting.com
Printed in the USA
JSHW020203050523
41295JS00002B/12

9 781936 657780